52 MOVEMENT
SNACKS

A CREATIVE HOW TO GUIDE
FOR INVITING MORE
MOVEMENT INTO YOUR LIFE

Trisha Durham

Trisha Durham

Cover design and illustrations by: Devin Timpone

Movement Snacks: A Creative How To Guide for Inviting More Movement Into Your Daily Life/ Trisha Durham. —1st ed.

ISBN 978-0-578-33351-9

CONTENTS

DEDICATION 4

TINY BOOK PREFACE....................5

WHAT IS A MOVEMENT SNACK 6

DEFINITIONS TO NOTE 8

WHY MOVEMENT SNACKS.............11

YOUR ACTIVITY LIST 13

DEAR HUMAN 15

52 MOVEMENT SNACKS 17

WHAT NOW..................................37

MOVEMENT SNACKS GO HERE 38

To Kelly for never skimping on the fun or the love. To my dad for driving me to every dance class and teaching me how to be curious.

This is a tiny book about a very important topic: Human movement. I wrote it because fitness culture can be exhausting and no book out there speaks enthusiastically about the power of moving your body in small, ordinary ways. In a world that is constantly pushing us onto the next complicated fitness fad please allow this book to be a reminder that you are once and always a mover.

Curious as a cloud. I've always been fascinated with how the human body can move and how physical activity helps us regulate our feelings and responses to the world we live in. I believe showing people how to add movement to their day can lead to more ways to feel present. More movement, more fun, more feeling good.

Never underestimate the big importance of small things. - The Midnight Library, Matt Haig

W hat is a movement snack? A movement snack is exactly what it sounds like. A small amount of physical activity is woven into the fabric of your day to help you recharge and remember you are more than your work, more than the roles you play. Movement snacks are a portal into a kind of playful awareness that our body and mind welcome, they can happen anywhere you are to help break up prolonged periods of sitting or inactivity. No gym or spandex required.

I've always enjoyed weaving small bits of movement whenever and wherever I can - while waiting for tea to steep, during commercial breaks, waiting for the light at a crosswalk. I've been known to do some yoga at the airport while waiting at the gate. It feels like a secret game I get to play with my environment. The idea is to provoke tiny moments of awareness. How can I move here? What can I do in this space besides what is expected from it? When you approach movement in this way it invites curiosity and creativity that makes you notice your surroundings. It's a simple way to implement mindfulness into your day. Physical activity, laughter and creativity are three ways to regulate the nervous system and complete the stress cycle. Additionally, it is the small movements, the foundational moves: squat, lunge, hinge, push, pull, reach and rotation that add up to being able to do the bigger dynamic moves often required for sports and fitness classes. The little things really do add up.

Once you start doing movement snacks, you'll find more places and opportunities to do them. Hooray, let's move.

Much more of the brain is devoted to movement than to language. Language is only a little thing sitting on top of this huge ocean of movement. - Oliver Sacks.

For clarity's sake it's worth noting the difference between these similar but different words: physical activity, exercise and movement.

Physical activity: is any movement that requires energy and is carried out by skeletal muscles.

Exercise: is by definition, planned, structured, repetitive and intentional movement where improvement or maintenance of physical fitness is an objective. Exercise is a subcategory of physical activity. All exercise is physical activity, but not all physical activity is exercise.

Movement: Often used interchangeably with the words physical activity and exercise, movement however, differs in that the human body and its many systems can move and change shape beyond our voluntary requests. For example, goose bumps are considered movement albeit a type of involuntary movement. Physical activity and exercise are movement, but not all movement is physical activity and exercise.

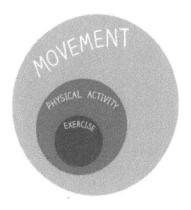

Remember that exercise isn't the only way to be active. You can make movement happen by building it into your day rather than it being this separate thing that you have to do at a designated time and place for a specific duration.

Play is also a relevant word to the topic of movement. Play is most often linked to children, but play theorist and researcher, Brian Sutton-Smith argued that any useful definition of play must apply to both adults and children.

That's because play can happen at any life stage and is present in many mammals and birds. Play helps diminish consciousness of self. We stop thinking about the fact that we are thinking. Play sparks creativity, joy and curiosity which sets us up to stress less and learn more. For these reasons you'll find some of the movement snacks in this book include elements of play.

WHY MOVEMENT SNACKS?

1. Because driving to a gym or yoga studio isn't always possible.

2. Because 60 minutes or nothing leaves a lot of people out of the fitness equation.

3. Because movement snacks invite awareness, creativity and play. Yay.

4. Because moving (and not moving) adds up over days, weeks, months and years.

5. Because snacks provide a boost of energy that help us live, work, focus and play.

6. Because taking a few minutes during the day to move thoughtfully helps land you in the present moment by bringing you back home to your body.

7. Because movement can fix a lot of things - our mood, our energy and our body. Every system in our body relies on movement to function. Movement is how we keep our cells happy, healthy and nourished.

8. Our brains love variety and variability.

Rest in reason and move in passion - Kahlil Gabon

We are walking hearts and nervous systems. Current estimates are that there are 30-50 trillion cells in the human body. And each of those cells is constantly adapting to your current lifestyle to make you more efficient for the tasks you do most often. This is perhaps one of the most exciting and useful things to understand about the human body. We truly are a use it or lose it being.

We may think of exercise as the gold standard, but the reality is everything we do and everything we DON'T do is shaping our ability to move. It's not that you are out of shape, it's that you are in shape for the things you do most frequently. Said another way, the body adapts to the loads and positions you spend the most time in. And around and around it goes. Going to a fitness class or returning to a physical activity you haven't done in a long time can feel daunting if you haven't been actively moving your body. The good news is anyone, regardless of age or ability can improve their capacity to move if they are willing to work at it.

To get clear on how you are moving about your environment make a list of all the physical activity you do in a typical day. This will give you a fascinating look at all the simple and mundane ways you are moving or not moving your body. Don't include things like blinking your eyes, though that is technically movement. But do include physical activity like yard work, walking to the curb to fetch the mail, carrying a child in your arms and folding laundry. Include the positions you find yourself in the most. For example, sitting or standing at your job x number of hours.

If your list is short, don't fret. Turn judgement into curiosity and use it as a starting point to discover all the ways you can add movement snacks into your day.

Movement Snacks

_____
_____
_____
_____
_____
_____
_____
_____
_____
_____
_____
_____
_____
_____
_____
_____
_____
_____
_____
_____
_____
_____
_____
_____
_____
_____
_____

Dear lovely human reading this, you don't need special clothing or fancy studio equipment to move your body. You have permission, a standing invitation that never expires to bring movement into your day, no matter where you're at. Start to notice the moments in-between and you'll surely find there's space and time to move your body.

If you wait until you're in a gym or on a yoga mat to move your body you may very well miss out on physical activity altogether. You don't have to do prescriptive or hard punishing exercise for your movement to count, or for it to be useful. As Dr. Colleen Reichamann is noted for saying, In order to rediscover the joy of movement we must stop asking if our exercise counts.

What's clear is that all the things that make up your awesome life plus a thousand other things will get in the way. As you begin this new snack size way of viewing movement it may help to schedule it on your phone or paper calendar. Make a two minute appointment. Don't cancel.

Each of the movement snacks in the pages that follow are to be carried out properly and with care. Honor your limits. It is possible to modify them, combine them and invent new ones.

52 MOVEMENT SNACKS TO GET YOU GOING

1. Stand on one leg and brush your teeth, wash your favorite coffee mug, moisturize your face.

2. Sit on the floor more. Ok, technically not movement, but the floor is a location we don't spend as much time on now that we have cozy furniture to hold us up. Sitting on the floor requires your core to hold you up and your legs and hips to move in delightfully different ways that couches and chairs do not.

3. Shoulder flossing. Hold each end of a scarf or a belt in your hands. Raise your arms overhead behind you and back again. Floss daily. Enjoy the stretch. It's my go to move for knocking the rust off the shoulders

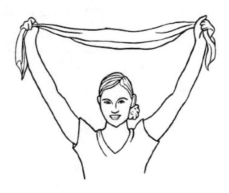

4. Take the stairs as often as possible. This is one of the simplest ways to include more physical activity into your day and requires little if any extra thought.

5. Spend more time barefoot. Your feet are your foundation and they need to move too. Free them from your shoes. Can you spread all your toes apart? Can you move your big toe independently from your other toes? Spending 3 minutes working on your feet can be its own mindful meditation.

6. Arm swinging. The best way to shake off the day. Just like it sounds. Use as little effort as possible. Stand with feet hip distance apart. Turn your body side-to-side. Allow your arms to come along for the ride.

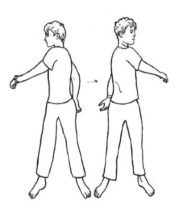

7. Leg swinging. Stand on one leg. Swing the other leg forward and back. Lots of momentum, not so much effort from the swinging leg. Hold onto a wall or chair for support.

8. At home circuit. Place a pillow, pile of laundry or stack of books on the floor to use as an obstacle you can step, squat, or jump over. Baby gates work too! How else can you use an ordinary household object to create an interesting physical activity?

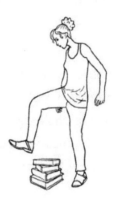

9. Take yourself for a walk. You need to be let out too. A tiny walk, a short walk. It all counts.

10. Do five jumping janes. How about five more?

11. Stepping stones. A movement snack for high play, balance and agility. Two versions of this to accommodate your location - out and about OR from home:

   • Look down and identify a pattern on the floor or sidewalk and choose to only step on a certain color or shape.

   • Set up yoga blocks, books, pillows or pieces of paper on the floor to serve as your stepping stones. Arrange in a simple straight line or challenge yourself by placing the "stones" further apart. Once walking is easy, try crawling.

12. Stand up during commercials, between zoom calls, in waiting rooms, after lunch. Flip the phrase, *take a load off*. Instead take a load ON. This is especially helpful for those who otherwise sit a lot.

13. Teacup drills. One of my favorite ways to knock the rust off the shoulders. Hold a book flat in your palm without using your fingers to grip or hold it. Begin to move your arm and explore all the possible ways you can move without dropping the book. Notice how your wrist, elbow and shoulder work together to keep the book upright while you move your arm. Repeat with the other arm. Mobility is served.

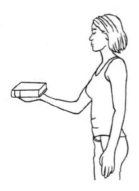

14. Draw figure eights with just your index finger, then your elbow, your whole arm. Now stand on one leg and draw those figure eights with your foot, your ankle, your whole leg.

15. Get up and down from the floor in as many different ways you can think of. There's no wrong way to do it. When this gets easier, try getting up and down without using your hands.

16. Have an old hand weight or kettlebell collecting dust in the corner? Bring it out into your living/work space so when your eyes land on it you can pick it up and walk around the room with it, hold it overhead, squat with it. It doesn't have to be a whole workout session. View your living space as a place where movement can happen.

17. Wax on, wax off standing leg circles. Stand on one leg. Lift your other leg up with a bent knee, circle that leg out to the side and lower to stand on it going onto the other leg.

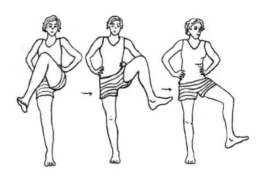

18. Raise your arms overhead. Really reach up and let your shoulders lift up too. Circle your hands and wiggle your fingers while you're up there. When was the last time you raised both your arms overhead? Sometimes it's the simple moves that disappear from our daily routine. It's a good day to invite them back in.

19. Find a straight line, lay out a tailor's tape or long piece of ribbon and walk it like you are on a balance beam or a tightrope, whichever you prefer to envision. Can you walk it backwards?

20. Hip dips. Stand on one leg sideways on a step, curb, book or yoga block, with legs straight, hike your hip up and down. Switch the standing leg and do the other side.

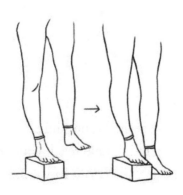

21. Get low and crawl. Crawling uses all four limbs and is one of the first forms of locomotion we do as infants. If crawling sounds like your jam - try out these other variations: bear crawl (or down dog crawl), crab crawl, belly crawling.

22. Do an incline pushup at your kitchen counter. Place your hands on the counter then walk your feet back until you feel some of your body weight is in your arms and your body is in a diagonal line. Either hold plank or try a few push ups this way.

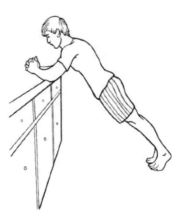

23. Do a yoga (half) sun salutation. Start by standing tall. Inhale reach your arms overhead, exhale fold forward, inhale lift

halfway up, exhale fold forward, inhale rise to standing.

24. Squat more. If you are new to squatting, start using a chair, feet planted wide. Stand up and sit down five times. Squat while you're waiting for your coffee or tea to steep.

25. Take five mindful breaths. You don't have to change or fix or do anything special with it. Just notice where your body moves when you breathe. Place your hands around your ribs or waist to invite more awareness to the experience. Breathing is movement. Breathing is core work at its essence.

26. Halfway! What's your favorite movement snack so far? We're more likely to keep doing the things we enjoy most. Identify 3-5 of your favorites from this list and combine them into one big snack. write them down and put them on your refrigerator. Do them whenever you catch a glimpse of the list.

27. Park your car farther away from the store entrance (on purpose) and enjoy the extra steps.

28. Cat-cow pose. Get down onto your hands and knees into a table top shape. Arch and round your spine like a wave. Feel everything between head and tailbone move.

29. Swimmers and windmills. Two things not usually seen together until we think about them in the context of your shoulders.

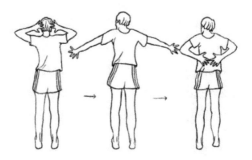

- First the swimmers: From standing or seated, put your hands behind your head like you would for a sit-up. Keep elbows wide as you open your arms, lowering them to bring them behind your low back. That's the move. Find the flow and do as many as it takes for your shoulders to feel warm and roomy.

- Now the windmills. Similar to the swimmers, but different. Start with one hand behind your head, the other behind your back - alternate each arm from head to low back.

30. Spinal twist. Can be done seated in a chair at your desk or standing using a wall for support and leverage. Breathe while you hold the twist for a few moments. Repeat other side.

31. Place your hand on a wall, keep it there and find all the ways you can move around and under it. Let this constraint spark that creative playful vibe.

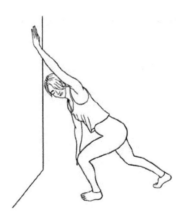

32. Do child's pose, puppy pose, down dog pose. Use these yoga poses as a way to expose your body to new shapes and positions that they may not otherwise get to be in.

33. Lift a bottle of laundry detergent, bag of cat food, or a 12 pack of sparkling water over your head. No hand weights, no problem. This movement snack gets you lifting more than the weight of your own arm overhead. Once you start doing this, you can no longer say, *I don't lift weights*.

34. Roll around on the floor. Get back to basics by laying on the floor, belly down and rolling over. It's a developmental move we learn as babies that lays the core groundwork for moving well in dynamic ways. Try initiating the roll with your arm and then with your leg.

35. Windshield wiper your hips. Sit in a chair or on the floor and lean back into your hands. With knees bent and feet anchored wide, slowly move your knees side to side.

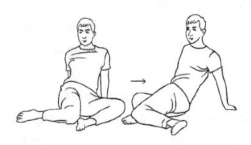

36. Stand on one leg while you're waiting in line at the grocery store, coffee shop, taco stand. It's a simple sneaky way to engage in balance and make your wait time more interesting.

37. Let's hang. Hanging is one of the best feeling moves that adults don't do a lot of. Holding onto an overhead bar will improve your grip strength and is said to be great for overall shoulder health. In my own personal experience with hanging it makes me feel strong, stretched and awake. You can incorporate hanging into your routine by placing a pull-up bar in one of your home doorways. Every time you pass through, reach up and hang. Start by keeping your feet on the ground until you feel strong enough to lift one or both of them off. Another way is the horizontal hang. Hold onto a secure doorknob or crown molding and lean out away from it - this too is hanging. Locate a neighborhood playground as there are always options for hanging there.

38. Hip circles. Stand with hands on your hips and your feet hip distance apart. Circle your hips as if you were hula hooping. Make the biggest, most thorough circle possible. Now

reverse the circle and go the other way. Try it slow, try it fast. Notice what you notice.

39. Legs up a wall. Locate open wall space and get into the pose by lying on your back and arranging your legs vertically up the wall. Your head, back and tailbone remain on the floor. Your body makes an L shape. For extra support use a rolled up towel beneath your tailbone. This pose can also be done with legs bent at a 90 degree angle to rest on chair seat. Feel your whole body in this shape. Be as present as you can considering how little time we spend with our legs in the air above our head.

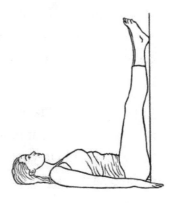

40. Jumping and heel thrumming. Jump up and down on both feet, then jump on one foot. Now try jumping with your eyes closed. If your feet and legs are new to jumping and not ready to leave the ground then try to bend and re-straighten your knees as quickly as you can while keeping the heels down. As you straighten your legs as if to jump, allow your heels to lift. Baby steps, er baby jumps. An alternative to jumping is heel thrumming: stand on both feet, lift and lower your heels rapidly, be purposefully heavy in your heels as you lower so that you can feel the reverb of the floor. Jumping helps supply more blood and oxygen to your muscles and is good for balance and coordination. It's also considered a functional move which is the type of fitness we can use in our daily living.

41. Go for a Skip. Skipping is fancy fun jogging, and it's good for your brain. Skip through a crosswalk, skip to your car, skip to the corner and back. Skip across the room you are in.

42. Fill a book bag with canned goods or other household items until it feels heavy, but still possible to lift. Now squat, lunge, lift and move in all the ways. No dumbbells, no problem.

43. Put your socks and shoes on standing up. A fun and simple way to include both balance and mobility into your daily routine. Stand near your bed for extra support in case you need to bail. At the end of the day do this in reverse - take your socks and shoes off standing up.

44. Standing mountain climbers. Place your hands on a wall, countertop or your desk. Walk your feet back till you're on a slight incline. High march your knees AKA mountain climbers.

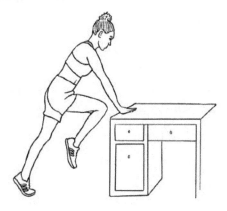

45. Find the nearest window to look out or go outside and gaze as far off into the distance as you can. See how many different objects you can identify. With all the up close screen gazing we do, our eyes need dynamic movement and rest too.

46. Take a mindful golf swing. Come into a golfer's stance ready to swing your invisible club. Keep your eyes on your hands as you slowly wind up and swing. This is a simple way to move your whole body including your eyes, head and vestibular system.

47. Rub (clean) hands together vigorously, then cover your eyes and face with cupped hands. Close your eyes. Block out the world for a moment and give your eyes a rest.

48. Let's play! The floor is lava, gluten, patriarchy, insert your desired thing to avoid and go about moving around the space you're in. Your need for play doesn't end once you're an adult. Play can positively impact your nervous system by improving your ability to self regulate and maintain your sense of calm amidst life's demands. When you're feeling stuck and disconnected, play can help get you out of your head and back into your body.

49. Stand on one leg and reach your other foot as far out in front of you as you can. Like you're dipping your big toe into water. Explore reaching out into all the different directions like the numbers on a clock: 12, 3, 6, 9. For more of a balance challenge, try this while standing on a yoga block or book.

50. Find a handrail, banister or similar structure that you can duck under and step over. Do that as many times as you can till someone looks at you and smiles.

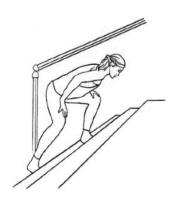

51. Move your spine in all of its six directions. Right and left side bend, right and left twist, forward fold and back bend.

52. Rock your body. From tabletop position (hands and knees) lean forward into your hands, then rock back into your heels. Now you're rocking. This dynamic version of rocking can help relieve that stiff feeling in your hips and improve mobility. Bonus: rocking initiates a calming effect in the parasympathetic nervous system.

By no means is this list exhaustive, but I hope these 52 movement snacks spark your curiosity and broaden your options for physical activity. I hope you find yourself asking, how can I move here? Borrow my favorite prompt: #whatmovesme

WHAT NOW?

Keep going. Keep noticing. Keep walking, skipping, jumping, squatting, sliding, twisting, swinging, hanging, playing, lunging, folding, bending, crawling, climbing, waving, kicking, hopping, slinking, rolling, flossing, reaching, circling, hula-ing, dancing, pushing, pulling, hauling, lifting, carrying, grooving, balancing, wiggling, grooving. Feel and deal. You've made your way through the 52 snacks, you're making time and space to move your body. What new way can you move?

Give new meaning to the phrase *take a break*. Break up long periods of inactivity with a movement snack. When it comes to physical activity and exercise, you are more likely to keep doing the things you enjoy most. Here are two extra pages where you can write down your favorite movement snacks or invent your own.

MOVEMENT
SNACKS GO HERE
↓

_____
_____
_____
_____
_____
_____
_____
_____
_____
_____
_____
_____
_____
_____
_____
_____
_____
_____
_____
_____
_____
_____
_____
_____
_____
_____
_____

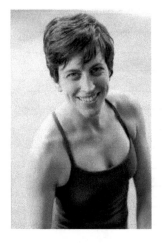

Trisha Durham is a multi-passionate movement educator and fitness trainer who writes. Her mission is to help people move more comfortably, kindly and competently. She gleefully smashes harmful fitness myths that get in the way. This is her first book. She lives online at www.trisha.yoga.

CPSIA information can be obtained
at www.ICGtesting.com
Printed in the USA
LVHW021629191122
733280LV00028B/2291